PROPER
BENCH PRESS FORM

The Beginner's Guide to Warm-Up, Technique, and Injury Prevention

Nicholas Gallo, PT, DPT

TABLE OF CONTENTS

———

INTRODUCTION

I have written this guide to help people learn the essential bench press technique that was not taught to me when I began weight training. Whether you are an absolute beginner or have some experience weight lifting, I know that you will find this helpful. Just a little background information about me: the first time I started lifting weights was in high school. I remember that I absolutely hated it the first time I tried it. I knew absolutely nothing about it and was very bad at it. I felt like I was completely lost, and one exercise really intimidated me: The Bench Press. I saw all those stronger people lifting more weight than I. I was embarrassingly weak at it. As I began lifting more and more, I improved in strength. However, after a while, things began to hurt and I began to have some aches in my shoulders and other areas. What I did not realize was that I was making critical errors that were allowing this to happen.

After receiving my undergraduate degree, I pursued a doctorate in Physical Therapy. I am currently a board-certified Doctor of Physical Therapy. During my time in school, I learned extensively about human anatomy and how body mechanics greatly affect results. I began to apply these principles to my own body and started to improve the way that I weight train. I have applied these principles to my bench press routine and assigned them to people who have come to me with injuries.

After graduating from Physical Therapy School, I began to treat individuals who had injured themselves bench pressing. These injuries spanned from wrist, shoulder, neck, etc. I'd always ask, "How is your form?" They would show me their forms and there was always something incorrect about it. The bar would be placed in the wrong position in their hands, the bar would be lowered incorrectly, things of that nature. Or people would have muscular imbalances in their body, such as rotator cuff weakness, lack of shoulder mobility, etc. Therefore, if the bench press is an exercise that people want to get back to, I find myself reviewing this a lot. During my time treating these individuals I began to fine-tune these improvements to myself. Through trial and error I have found a successful step-by-step process to accomplish optimal, pain-free form.

Another thing I wish I had learned more about in the beginning of my weightlifting career is the importance of warming up and stretching afterwards. If your muscles are not properly warmed up and ready to complete a lift, they will not function correctly. Fradkin et al. determined that, "This analysis has shown that performance improvements can be demonstrated after completion of adequate warm-up activities, and there is little evidence to suggest that warming-up is detrimental to sports participants." This means that if you are warming up correctly, you will notice athletic improvements and no adverse effects, which in my experience is true. Therefore, in this publication I will go over some of the key warm-up exercises I recommend to people. These exercises include beneficial things for the shoulders, upper back, and other parts of the body. I also go over technique, step by step, for bench pressing, going in depth on correct setup and form. I not only will do this for the barbell bench press, but I also include some ideal tips for other variations such as dumbbell bench press and whether you want to vary the bench angle. Finally, I include some essential stretching and mobility exercises that I have people use to cool down. This is important for several reasons, but in my experience it helps people, including myself, stay injury free.

In this publication I will show you how to evaluate your bench press form, how to warm up properly, and some injury prevention techniques you can do each workout. As we get older, it's important to not only maintain strength but also mobility in our joints and flexibility in our muscles in order to stay pain free. Therefore, I will also explain some tests to determine if you have muscle imbalances and weaknesses hindering your bench press ability. It also helps a person maintain optimal posture. If you feel like your posture is suffering, my publication *Posture Pain: Key Strategies to Stay Pain Free at Your Desk and in Life* goes into great depth on this topic.

Finally, I would like to point out that I offer free educational videos showing a variety of different treatments and diagnoses on my YouTube channel *Physical Therapy 101*. This channel was started to provide free, to-the-point exercises to patients and practitioners. This channel is continuously being updated and provides a slew of information spanning several diagnoses, so please subscribe if you are interested. Supplemental information can be found on our website www.physicaltherapy101.net.

1

WARMING UP

Can You Do 10 Push-Ups?

The Bench Press is a very advanced exercise that you should not rush into with poor form. There is one test that I recommend to people and that is, can you perform 10 push-ups maintaining optimal form? If you can perform 10 body weight push-ups while maintaining great form, then yes, you have a good base to begin bench pressing. I do, however, want you to try this, and I will go over the correct push-up form even if you believe you can already do it. Learning this is beneficial because when you do a push-up with optimal form, you are learning the optimal form for bench pressing.

First off, when you go into a push-up position, you want your hands to be at shoulder width, or preferably a little bit wider. Your hands should be directly under your shoulders. Most people do those two steps correctly. Let's focus on head positioning for a second. A lot of times I see that a person's head will come forwards and put a lot of strain on the neck. It's important to make sure that your head remains in line with your shoulders, if you were to look at yourself from the side. Now, I will say that depending on who you talk to, they prefer that you look forward as you do push-ups. From an injury prevention standpoint and for the sake of perfecting this motion to bench press correctly, I would not recommend that here.

Now let's look at your shoulder position. Are you shrugging your shoulders up towards your head, or are they down? You want to make sure that your shoulders stay down, a popular cue I like to use is, "Tuck your shoulder blades into your back pockets." If you keep your shoulders shrugged upwards, you are putting yourself at right for a shoulder injury.

As you descend and go towards the ground, your elbows will bend and go out from the side of your body. A big mistake I see often is that as a person is doing push-ups, their elbows will really flare out from the sides, which puts tremendous strain on the shoulders. A good rule of thumb to aim for is, as you descend to the ground, try to maintain a 45-degree angle from your elbows to your body.

As you move further down the body, common mistakes that I see are that people allow their hips to sag and their back to arch. In order to prevent this, I give people a cue to engage their core. I commonly tell them, "Try to pull your belly button toward your spine." Doing this engages a muscle known as the Transversus Abdominis and creates a rigid spine. Another key thing to do is to engage your glutes. "Try to squeeze your butt cheeks together," is a cue I give for this.

If you have the ideal setup and are following all of these directions I have given above, it's time to try 10 push-ups. I see a lot of people that rush through these, which is good if you are going for speed, but it is often at the expense of optimal form. Maintaining optimal form, I like to descend towards the ground at a count of "1 Mississippi," and raise up at a count of "1 Mississippi." This is a good amount of time that shows you have control.

Bench Press Warm-Up

You can do 10 push-ups with optimal form and are almost ready to do the bench press. One thing I see commonly is that people are not warming up properly. What many people don't realize is that the Bench Press can be very risky for your shoulders if they are not warmed up/strengthened properly. The area of the shoulder that can be injured during this exercise is commonly known as the Rotator Cuff. It's a group of four small muscles: Teres Minor, Infraspinatus, Supraspinatus, and Subscapularis. These muscles all have individual actions, but their main function is to work as a unit to stabilize the shoulder. If you have very weak stabilization at the shoulder joint, then you are not only limited in the amount of weight you are able to lift, but you are also putting yourself at a HUGE risk for injury.

There is another area that I like to include in the warm-up: the Scapula, also known as the Shoulder Blade. A lot of the movement at the shoulder depends on scapular motion; therefore, some of these exercises also include scapular motion. The scapula is extremely important, especially when dealing with posture. Kim et al. determined in a study that, "These findings suggest that the elastic band exercise program used in the study is effective for lengthening the pectoralis major and correcting rounded shoulder and forward head posture." This means that with the regular use of elastic bands in their study, people were able to correct their posture with simple band exercises. Since ideal posture helps prevent injury in the bench press, this warm-up routine will target exactly that.

To begin warming up, do 10 minutes of cardiovascular training just to get the blood flowing. I personally jog on a treadmill or do some type of jump roping. Anything to get things moving and to feel more limber. Next, what I like to do and what I recommend for people is to grab a resistance band. All resistance bands are different and their color scheme refers to different resistances, so I recommend that you choose a very easy one to begin with.

Band Pull Aparts - Palms Down

The first exercise that I like to begin with is known as the Band Pull Apart with the palms down. I really like this exercise because it focuses mainly on the scapular motion I was referring to earlier and strengthens the upper back, which most people are deficient in. It is also providing some activation for areas in the back of the shoulder, which is often overlooked in weight lifting.

1. To begin, grip a resistance band straight in front of you with your palms facing downward at approximately shoulder width. Allow your shoulders to round slightly. You want your elbows

completely straight in this position, with no bend in your arms.

2. Now, as the name suggests, you want to pull the band apart by moving your hands out laterally to your sides while maintaining straight elbows.

3. As you are moving your arms to your sides, you want to be sure that you are pinching your shoulder blades. I commonly say, "As if you are trying to hold a pencil between them," as a cue.

4. Pull the band apart until it touches your mid chest and then allow the band to come back to the starting position under control.

When you round the shoulders during this exercise, it allows your shoulder blades to perform a motion known as protraction. As you pull the band apart, you want to squeeze your shoulder blades together. Squeezing the shoulder blades together allows your scapulas to perform a motion known as retraction. Just like the push-up form, you want to make sure that you are not shrugging your shoulders toward your head while you perform the exercise. Another common mistake people make is that they are doing these too fast and not controlling the band. It is recommended to do 10-15 repetitions of this exercise.

Band Pull Aparts - Palms Up

The next exercise is nearly the same as the previous one, except your palms are now facing the ceiling.

1. To begin, grip the resistance band straight in front of you with your palms facing upward at

approximately shoulder width. Allow your shoulders to round slightly. You want your elbows completely straight in this position, with no bend in your arms.

2. Like the prior exercise, pull the band apart by moving your hands out laterally to your sides and maintaining straight elbows.

3. Be sure to pinch the shoulder blades as you are moving your arms out to the sides.

4. Pull the band apart until it touches your mid chest and then allow the band to come back to the starting position under control.

When you perform this variation, you are allowing your shoulders to do a motion known as external rotation, which is a function of the Teres Minor and Infraspinatus of the Rotator Cuff. Therefore, with this exercise you are not only warming up your scapulas, but you are also providing some great rotator cuff strengthening. It is recommended to do 10-15 repetitions of this exercise.

Band Pull Aparts - Overhead

Another band pull apart exercise I like to do is virtually the same as the top two except, instead of starting with the band straight out in front of you, it is now overhead and slightly forward.

1. To begin, grip the resistance band with your palms facing upward at approximately shoulder width. You want your elbows completely straight in this position with no bend in your arms.

2. Now, as I mentioned before, you want the starting position of the band to be overhead and slightly forward.
3. Next, you will move your arms to your sides like in the prior two exercises.
4. Be sure to be pinching your two shoulder blades together like in the prior two exercises.
5. Pull the band apart until it touches your upper chest and then allow the band to come back to the starting position under control.

This exercise works on a motion known as scapular depression when you are lowering the band and scapular elevation when you are allowing it to return to the starting position. When you pull the band towards your body, you are activating a muscle known as the Lower Trapezius, which is often overlooked in training. This muscle being deficient can cause the scapula to move abnormally and lead to problems. Like before, it is recommended to do 10-15 repetitions of this exercise.

No Money - Palms Up

This next exercise is known commonly as the "No Money" exercise. It focuses on a shoulder motion known as external rotation that most people are weak with.

1. To begin, bend your arms so that they are both making a 90-degree angle.
2. Now grab the resistance band with your palms facing up.

3. Rotate your hands outward, away from each other, while you pinch your shoulder blades together and down. Be sure to maintain contact with your elbows to your body.

4. Then allow the band to come back to the starting position under control.

If you are doing this exercise correctly, you will feel tiny muscles burning in the back of your shoulders and shoulder blades. A common mistake is that as a person fatigues, their elbows are not against their body. Be sure to keep them in contact with your sides for maximum activation of the proper muscles. It is recommended to do 10-15 repetitions of this exercise.

Shoulder External Rotation With Band

This is an isolation exercise that targets the same area that was working in the previous exercise; however, instead of both arms working at once, you will work one at a time.

1. To start, anchor a resistance band by either closing it in a door or by tying it to something stable.

2. To strengthen the right arm, your left side will be facing the end of the band anchored. You will be gripping the band in your right hand with it.

3. For the starting position, your right arm should be across your body.

4. Next, you will move your right arm out to the side like you did in the prior exercise, maintaining your right elbow touching your side.

5. Then allow the band to come back to the starting position under control.
6. After you complete a set of 10-15 repetitions, switch the band to the other hand and complete the same steps.

This is a great isolation exercise because you are working one arm at a time and not allowing the stronger side to compensate for the weaker one.

Shoulder Internal Rotation With Band

This is another great isolation exercise; however, you are doing the opposite motion of the prior exercise.
1. To start, anchor a resistance band by either closing it in a door or by tying it to something stable.
2. To strengthen the right arm, your right side will be facing the end of the band anchored. You will be gripping the band in your right hand with it.
3. For the starting position, your right hand should be directly in front of you, gripping the band.
4. Next, you will move your right arm toward the inside of your torso with the arm across your body.
5. Then allow the band to come back to the starting position under control.
6. After you complete a set of 10-15 repetitions, switch the band to the other hand and complete the same steps.

Internal rotation is another action completed by the rotator cuff muscle Subscapularis; therefore, I like this exercise to get that muscle engaged and warmed up.

Serratus Push-Ups

The final exercise that I recommend for people to warm up with is known as a Serratus Push Up. This exercise is done by maintaining the same optimal push-up form I went over earlier, but there is a slight variation to include the Serratus Anterior, which is an often overlooked muscle. Its primary function is to help the scapula maintain an optimal position during movement. If this muscle is not properly included in your training regimen, it can lead to a condition known as Scapular Winging.

1. To begin, go into the correct push-up position as before.
2. While you descend to the ground, pinch your shoulder blades together.
3. As you press to the top of the push-up, allow your shoulder blades to separate and allow your shoulders to round forward.
4. Complete this for 10 repetitions.

This exercise does not only warm up your Serratus Anterior muscles, but it also allows your chest and other bench press muscles to warm up. If this exercise becomes too difficult when you include the movements of the Serratus Anterior, you can start by performing this exercise on your elbows. If you do this on your elbows, be sure to still follow the correct push-up setup.

2

THE BENCH PRESS EXERCISE

Barbell Bench Press Safety

Now that I have gone over warm-ups and you can perform the 10 push-ups with optimal form, I will go into detail on the correct form for the Bench Press Exercise. It may seem simple, but there are some key components that need to be addressed for you to stay injury free when performing this great exercise. Before I discuss this in depth, I want to say that I ALWAYS recommend having a spotter when performing this exercise in case you cannot lift it. If you get in a situation where you cannot lift the bar up off of your chest, it can lead to injury big time. I've seen videos of bars landing on people's necks, chest, faces, etc. These could all have been avoided if the person had simply used a spotter. If you do not want to use a spotter, I have seen people bench in the power rack, but for safety purposes I do not suggest it, especially if you are a beginner. Also, if you have a spotter, please make sure it is somebody who is paying attention! I can't tell you how many times I've seen people not pay attention and their friend injures themselves. Now let's get into the key components of the Bench Press. After each section I will include a summary of the key point so that it is easy to follow.

If you start to experience discomfort and are unsure what is causing it, I suggest going to a medical professional to be on the safe side. Take it from me, grinding through injuries is never a good thing and puts tremendous strain on your body. In prior years I remember that I did not want to stop bench pressing even though I had discomfort because I did not want to lose the strength that I had gained. As I became more educated on Physical Therapy and rehabilitation, I realized that if you push through injuries, you are setting yourself up for serious injury. The average recovery time for a rotator cuff tear surgery can be anywhere from four to six months and sometimes even longer, depending on the injury. It's not worth going through a surgery that can be prevented, so if you are experiencing sharp pains, rest and seek medical attention.

Pre-Lift Setup

Bar Setup

First and foremost, you want to make sure that the bar is in the middle of the bench and no longer on one side compared to the other. There will be instances when the bar is racked and it is uneven. Making sure that the bar is even on both sides allows the weight to be distributed evenly as you are lifting it. For example, if the bar is more towards the right compared to the left and you begin to lift it, you will overload the right side of your body, which can lead to injury.

Key Point: Check to see if the bar is even in the rack and not lopsided.

Grip Width

You are lying down and looking up at the bar. It is now time to determine your grip width. There are several variations to the grip width, as it is different for everybody. What I suggest, especially for beginners, is to pretend you have a bar in your hands and do the bench press motion. Just like the push-up, you want to make sure your elbows are not flaring out to 90 degrees at the sides. Usually, the comfortable width is somewhere near shoulder to a little more than shoulder width, but due to different body types this will vary. As a person has wider shoulders, their grip needs to be wider. If they have more narrow shoulders, then the grip needs to be more narrow. There is not a one size fits all for the grip width due to varying body sizes, but as long as you can prevent the elbows from flaring out, that is ideal. Also, it's important that your forearms are perpendicular to the floor at every position during the lift.

Key Point: Generally, shoulder width to slightly wider than shoulder width, depending on body type. You choose, as long as the elbows do NOT flare out to 90 degrees away from your body.

The Bar Grip

Gripping the bar is very important because if it is done wrong, it can be very painful to several body parts, including the wrist. Sometimes, what I see is that a person will grip the bar but it is too high in their hands. Gripping the bar too high on the hands can cause injury to your wrists because it places them in extreme wrist extension. You may have had a sprained wrist in the past where you tripped/slipped and put your hand out to brace yourself on the ground as you fell. This is a common way to injure the wrist, and when you do this bench pressing, it is no different. Placing the bar here results in the wrist being hyperextended and will lead to pain as you start adding more weight to the exercises. A good thing to remember is that you want your forearm and wrist to be in a complete straight line all the way down to your elbow. Therefore, the easiest way to accomplish this is by gripping the bar lower towards the wrist and not mid to upper palm.

The best way to set up your bench grip is to begin by placing the bar towards the bottom of your hand or at the base of your palm. Think of the bar as an extension of your forearm. You want both forearms to be straight forward pointing perpendicular to the ceiling and the bar to be resting this way as well. As the bar is resting there, wrap all your fingers except your thumb around the bar first. From here, I highly suggest wrapping your thumbs around the bar to hold it in place. Now, there are many different variations of gripping the bar for bench pressing, but I want you to know that I suggest this one because it is the safest. You will see people using thumbless grips and it may work for them. The method I am teaching you minimizes your risk of the bar slipping out of your hands and allows you to have a firm grip on the bar.

Now that you have four of your fingers around the bar, it's time to place the thumb around the bar as well.

With the thumb wrapped around you may see people that allow the thumb to rest on their index and middle fingers AND you may see people allowing the thumb to rest under the index finger. I suggest allowing the thumb to rest on top of the index and middle fingers because it allows less pressure to be added to the thumb.

Key Point: You should be gripping the bar close to the base of your palm. Make sure the thumb is wrapped around the bar for safety. Always make sure your wrists are straight and not bent during the lift to avoid wrist injuries.

Shoulder Blade Position

Now that you have the grip settled, it's important that I address the correct positions for your shoulder blades and your upper back. We did some warm-up exercises for this earlier because during the bench press you want your shoulder blades to be pinched together and down and back. I said earlier that you want to put them in your back pockets, which is the same cue I want you to use here. To make a more stable base, you also want to be pinching the shoulder blades together. I usually give a cue of, "Pinch your shoulder blades together as if you are trying to hold a pencil there." This provides stability and allows you to stick your chest out for greater activation while performing the lift. This will allow the chest to perform the majority of the work and decrease the load on the shoulders. It also decreases the distance that the bar will need to travel during the lift and make it easier than lifting with a flat chest.

Key Point: Keep shoulders back and shoulder blades pinched together for stability. Push your chest out for greater chest activation.

Back Arch

As you are setting up the lift and you squeeze your shoulder blades together, your back will naturally curve. A good cue to think about is that you want to be able to fit a hand under your back while you are bench pressing. Now, you will see powerlifters who arch their backs excessively in order to lift maximum loads on the bench press. They are doing this so that they can dramatically decrease the distance the bar has to travel so they can complete the lift. They put their spines in a position known as extension. If you do too much extension at your spine, you are really compressing things in your spinal column, which can lead to pain. Therefore, I do not suggest this unless you are a powerlifter.

Key Point: DO NOT OVERARCH. Maintain proper shoulder and shoulder blade position to create the natural arch of the spine.

Lower Body

Yes, the Bench Press is a great upper body exercise, but you want to make sure your lower body is not dormant during the lift! Just like the push-up, it is important to have your glutes engaged. A good way to do this is by having your feet flat on the floor. A good cue to remember is having your feet directly under your knees. Ideally, you want your shins to be perpendicular to the ceiling. If your feet are too far out, you don't have much pushing power from them and you are not nearly as stable. Now, you may see a powerlifter place their feet differently than this, and that is an advanced position. For our sake, however, it's a good idea to have them directly under the knees. When you are doing the actual lift of the bench press, you will be squeezing your glutes together just like during the push-ups we went over earlier. By doing this you are providing a very stable base for your lower body during the lift. You want to make sure that your butt does not come off the bench while you are doing this. This is considered cheating and is not nearly as stable. As the bar touches your chest, you want to drive through your feet and keep the glutes tight. This provides some extra stability and force as the bar is moving upwards.

I also want to mention that you will see people with their feet resting on the bench and sometimes even in the air while they are bench pressing. The rationale for this is that, if you are really beginning to arch your lower back excessively, this will help mitigate that. The benefit is that when your feet are not on the floor, your back will flatten on the bench and prevent this arching. This makes perfect sense; however, completely flattening your back may make other aspects of lifting properly more difficult, such as proper shoulder blade positioning and overall stability. Still, this is a great way to bench press if a person starts to experience lower back pain when their spine arches.

Key Point: Keep feet flat on the floor and shins pointing vertically so that they are perpendicular to the ceiling.

Make sure that your glutes are engaged and you are driving through the floor but keep your butt on the bench. If arching your back hurts, try with your feet on the bench or in the air.

The Actual Lifting

Breathing

Before you perform the lifting part, I want to go over an overlooked aspect of weight lifting: how to breathe correctly. Breathing is very important when it comes to weightlifting and it is often done incorrectly. There are two portions of the lift: the eccentric portion and the concentric portion. The eccentric portion of the lift is when you are lowering the bar to your chest and the concentric portion is when you are pushing the bar away from your chest. For the bench press, the best way to breathe is inhaling during the eccentric portion of the lift and breathing out during the concentric portion of the lift. A cue I use for people is to imagine that as the bar is getting lower to your body, you are trying to breathe it in, and when you are pressing the bar up, you are trying to blow it away. If you are performing other lifting exercises, it is typically suggested to breathe in during the eccentric portion and out during the concentric portion. You MAY read or have heard about other breathing variations such as the Valsalva maneuver, which I will not discuss in depth. Essentially, it involves a person trying to forcefully exhale against their closed airway. This is not for everybody and there are certain contraindications for this, so I do not advise it.

Key Point: Inhale when the bar is descending towards your chest and exhale as the bar moves away from your chest.

The Bar Lift-Off

Now that you have followed the directions above, you are ready to lift the bar off of the rack and begin the lift. One thing that is important is to make sure that your elbows are locked completely straight as you perform this first step. You don't want any bend in them because as you are lifting the bar off, it may result in you losing the bar, which would cause it to fall on top of you. Earlier, I said that you want to start with the bar over your eyes, but as you lift the bar off, you want to make sure that you allow your arm to come slightly forward so that the bar is directly over your shoulders.

Key Point: Keep elbows locked straight and begin with the bar over the eyes. Before you descend, have the bar directly over your shoulders.

The Bar Path

This is a very important step that is often overlooked. You have the bar lifted off and it is now positioned properly over your shoulders. A lot of times, people will either lower the bar too high on their body or it won't travel in an optimal path. The Bench Press is already a difficult exercise, especially as you begin to add weight. The last thing you want to do is make it more difficult with a suboptimal bar path. Since the setup has the bar over your eyes, as you lift the bar off the rack, you want your arms to come forward slightly so that the bar is over your shoulders and upper back area. If you lower the bar too high on your chest, your elbows will flare out to 90 degrees and, like I mentioned earlier, this is setting you up for injury. Therefore, you want it in an optimal position to prevent this.

You will start with the bar directly over your shoulders and lower it down to your mid chest area. This allows the bar to travel in a diagonal line. As you press upwards, you want the bar to go along the same diagonal path. This is not only the best bar path because it is the most stable, but it also allows you to lift more weight. Now, you will read that there are other benefits to certain bar paths that people use. For the purpose of fundamentals, the bar path should follow this diagonal path. If you feel like experimenting with things such as a J curve, which essentially means that the bar moves but curves at certain points, then you are free to do so. Just know that your beginning position and the point you are lowering to essentially remain the same.

As you are lowering the bar, keep in mind that you want your forearms to stay completely vertical at every angle. Any deviation from this can set you up for injury. It's also very important that you remember to lower the bar with CONTROL. You want your muscles engaged when the weight is on its way down and on its way back up. If you go too fast, you risk the weight slamming into your chest, also known as "bouncing." This can not only be damaging to your chest, but it is also a way of cheating during this lift. Now, lifting with control does not mean benching extremely slowly either. It means just controlling the weight down and controlling the weight back up.

Key Point: The starting position should be with the bar over your shoulders. The bar is then lowered to your mid chest area and pressed back up to directly over your shoulders.

Bottom Position

As the weight comes down, you want to remember to let the bar touch your mid chest area. As soon as the bar touches your mid chest, press it back upwards so that it is directly over your shoulders again. There are different bench variations, and one is known as the "Pause Bench." When you do it this way, you are literally allowing the weight to pause when it is down touching your chest. This is typically how a bench press competition will work, but for our case, I am not suggesting you pause there. As soon as the bar touches, you should be ready to press it back up. Now, I am NOT saying that you should bounce the bar off of your chest. This is a recipe for disaster and you can probably find many YouTube videos of a person doing this. Bouncing the bar off of your chest places extreme stress on your sternum and can lead to bruising and other injuries. It is also very difficult to keep your body fully tight and braced for the lift when you are doing the bench press. Therefore, it is not recommended.

You may also see people that bench press, but they are not allowing the bar to come all the way down. I cannot stress this enough: it is important to work your muscles in their full range of motion. Bringing the bar down partially instead of all the way will not work the chest muscles maximally. If you cannot go down all the way, check to make sure the weight is not too heavy. If it begins to hurt your shoulders, re-evaluate your form and make sure that you are not using bad technique. When you reach the bottom position, be sure that your forearms are pointing vertically so that they are perpendicular with the ceiling. The same rule as before applies with the elbows: you want to make sure that they are not flared out to 90 degrees from the body to prevent shoulder injury.

Key Point: Allow the bar to touch your mid chest and then press it back up. Like before, the bar should be over your shoulders. Maintain a vertical forearm position and prevent the elbows from flaring out. They should be less than 90 degrees from the side of your body.

Dumbbell Bench Press

I have discussed the barbell version of the bench press so far, but you will definitely see it performed with dumbbells in the gym. I really like the dumbbell bench press because unlike using a barbell, your joints can move more freely because your hands are not fixed on one point. Because of this, however, dumbbell bench press will be very taxing on your shoulder stabilization muscles, which is a very good thing. Whether you want to perform barbell or dumbbell bench press, I wanted to tell you that your form should remain NEARLY IDENTICAL. The only thing that will vary is the setup because you no longer have a rack holding the bar for you.

How to set up the dumbbell bench press properly begins with you having a dumbbell of equal weight in both hands and resting on your thighs. Now, before you lie with your back on the bench, you want to move the dumbbells as close as you can to the crease in your hips. This is suggested because when you roll back, they are already as close to the correct starting position as possible. As you roll back, press the dumbbells up and have them in the same starting position as we had the barbell and complete the exercise maintaining the same principles as before.

In order to reach the starting position, you may see people lift their legs as they roll back to help them put the dumbbells into place. I like this because it will help the dumbbells move into the correct position with less effort. If you do this, make sure you don't become too unstable and fall off of the bench holding the dumbbells because briefly your feet will not have contact with the ground. Also feel free to have a spotter close by to help stabilize your arms if you have doubts.

When you have completed the set, I suggest lowering the weights to your chest and keeping your elbows close to your body. If you can, try to lower them back to your thighs and sit up simultaneously. This is not only safest for the shoulders, but it is also safer especially if people are around you. If you cannot do this, I suggest keeping the dumbbells close to your hips and lowering them to the floor with control. I have been in gyms before where I've seen people drop them very uncontrolled and nearly hit a bystander. Also, if you allow the dumbbells to slam onto the floor, you risk breaking them and/or being yelled at in the gym.

3

AFTER BENCH PRESSING

———

After you Bench Press (or do any exercise, for that matter), I really believe in stretching the muscles you have used. When you are lifting weights, you are contracting muscles, which causes them to shorten. Over time, if you do not stretch them out again, this can lead to pains and even poor posture. The muscles of the chest also have a function at the shoulder joint. Therefore, it's important to make sure that you are stretching out your chest and shoulders after the exercise. I also include some foam rolling/soft tissue work. All of these exercises should be done, but the order can vary.

Check Your Shoulder Mobility

Now that you have completed your bench press workout, it's important to look at the mobility of your shoulders. What I mean by this is that our joints are supposed to move pain free in all different types of planes. The Glenohumeral Joint is what most people refer to as the shoulder. It is the most mobile joint in the human body. Therefore, if you want to bench press correctly and safely, it is ideal to have a full or near full range of motion at this joint. Now, I am not saying that you cannot bench press if you have some limitations . What I am saying, however, is that if you continue to lift with limitations, over time you may start to develop issues. This is also a great way to identify areas you need to work on to increase your mobility to stay pain free. There are tests that I do in the clinic to determine this that few people will know outside of the clinical setting. Therefore, I will outline some mobility tests that I use so that you can determine if you have any of these limitations.

The first test I want you to try is to take your right hand and raise it overhead. While in this position, let your arm bend so that your palm is now touching the back of your neck. This is testing two motions, known as shoulder abduction and shoulder external rotation, which are both essential movements. Now I want you to do this with the opposite hand. Did you feel one side that was more difficult than the other? Do you feel pain or discomfort? If you did, then this might mean that one side is more limited than the other. I will go over some stretches and things later on how to try and fix it. I suggest at the very least doing this in front of a mirror so that you can visualize specifically where each hand touches.

The next test is performed by starting with your right hand down at your side. You will then reach behind your back and allow the back of your hand to rest on your spine. This might be more difficult to do because it is not a common motion to some people. This is testing your shoulder adduction and shoulder internal rotation. In my experience, it is more common to be limited in this position compared to the prior one. Personally, I know that I am more limited in this motion in my right shoulder because I was an overhead throwing athlete for many years. If you are or were an overhead throwing athlete, then you may notice this as well.

I just went over two tests for shoulder mobility that you can use to evaluate yourself depending on how it feels. Now I want to go over a test that will give you some objective data so you can measure it. Like I mentioned above, you want your right arm raised overhead and you want your arm to bend so that your palm is touching the back of your neck. Now AT THE SAME TIME, reach behind your back and up your spine with your LEFT arm with the back of your hand resting on your spine. Now without moving excessively, slide your hands as close as possible together. When you have reached a position where you cannot slide any further, measure the distance between your middle fingers. Now, if you can touch your fingers, then this is the ideal position. If you cannot, however (most people can't, myself included), you have some restriction in your joint and I suggest doing some shoulder mobility exercises that I will outline next.

Shoulder Dislocations

The first exercise is for overall shoulder mobility and is a favorite among a lot of professional powerlifters, bodybuilders, etc. This exercise is commonly referred to as "Shoulder Dislocations." Don't worry, you are not actually dislocating your shoulders when you perform it, but it is a great exercise for overall shoulder mobility. I have found success with it after the workout when my shoulders and body are warmed up, but some people prefer to use it as a warm-up. Whether you do it before or after your workout, this is a great exercise for overall shoulder mobility.

To perform this exercise you will need some type of stick. People commonly use a broom stick, but it can also be done with a stretch strap or a towel. Now, you will grab it with both hands in a wide grip with the palms facing downwards. You will hold the stick out in front of you, which is the starting position. The goal of this exercise is to maintain the same hand position on the stick throughout the entire motion.

1. Lift your arms above your head and raise the bar toward the ceiling. During this motion, you rotate your shoulder blades upward as the bar moves past your face.

2. Once the stick is overhead, you pinch your shoulder blades and externally rotate your shoulders to pull the stick down and behind your back, until the stick touches the back of your body.

3. Now that the stick is behind your body, you reverse the process from before. You will start by pinching your shoulder blades and raise your arms to raise the bar from behind your body, toward the ceiling.

4. Rotate the shoulder blades upward as the stick moves up past your neck to overhead.

5. Lower the stick out front to the starting position.

During this exercise, you want to make sure you maintain a straight spine and be careful not to arch your back excessively. Another common error is to bend your elbows; you want to make sure that your elbows are locked straight the entire time. If you notice that you cannot perform the entire range of motion, try using a wider grip with your hands. Finally, be sure not to go too fast with this exercise. You want a nice steady motion. If you want to make this exercise more difficult, slowly narrow your grip on the stick.

Shoulder Internal Rotation Stretch With a Towel

You may have identified some motions that are deficit on one side compared to the other, which is completely normal. Many people have imbalances. The important thing is to do some exercises in order to try and correct them. A great shoulder stretch that I recommend is the towel stretch:

1. To set up this stretch, you want to hold the towel in one hand and allow it to drape over your shoulder down your back. For example, if you are stretching your right shoulder, the towel should be placed over your left shoulder and be held in your left hand.
2. Reach behind your back with your right hand and grip the towel.
3. Gently pull the towel up and allow your right hand to move across and up your back towards your right shoulder. A gentle stretch should be felt in the front or side of your shoulder.

4. Once you feel a stretch in your shoulder, hold the position for 10 seconds, and then slowly release the stretch. This stretch should be performed 10 times. Do not push past sharp pains.
5. After this, perform it on the left side.

Upper Trapezius Stretch

The main muscle involved in shrugging your shoulders upward is the Upper Trapezius muscle. If this muscle is tight, it will not only make it difficult to keep your shoulder blades in the optimal position during the bench press, but it can also lead to pain over time. Since a lot of people have tightness here, I want to include a stretch for this to help keep the muscle flexible.

1. Begin by facing forward and keeping your head straight.
2. To stretch your right Upper Trapezius muscle, allow your head to tilt to the left without rotating it.
3. This stretch can be progressed by taking your left hand to pull your head further, but it is important to NOT overstretch.
4. Once you feel a stretch, hold this position for 30 seconds and do it 4 times.
5. After this, perform it on the left side.

This stretch can be further intensified if the inactive arm is holding on to something to make sure the shoulder stays down. For example, if you are stretching the right Upper Trapezius muscle, grab onto a weight or something to keep the shoulder down and complete the stretch. You will feel more of a stretch in the area, but like I mentioned before, be sure not to overstretch this muscle.

Doorway Chest Stretch

The main chest stretch that I suggest afterwards is the Door Stretch. I really do like this stretch. You perform it with a doorway because it really allows you to stretch the chest muscles very well. Since you have worked them after bench pressing, it is important to stretch them back out again once you are finished. If a doorway is unavailable, you can still perform this stretch with the corner of a room, but know that if you do this, you may not be able to stretch as far.

1. In a doorway, place your hands at the bottom of the doorway and lean forward keeping your head in line with your body.
2. Now place one foot forward and bend your front knee until a stretch is felt.
3. If you do not feel a stretch here, try to step further through the door.
4. During this stretch, people will commonly make the mistake of letting their head fall forward. This is bad posture. It is important to keep your head in line with the rest of your body.
5. To make this stretch more intense, you can raise your arms up on the door frame like you are signaling a Field Goal and repeat the steps above.

You should feel the muscles stretch in the front of your shoulders and chest area as you perform this. I usually suggest holding this stretch for 20-30 seconds and performing it 4 times.

Posterior Shoulder Stretch

I want to also include a stretch for the back of the shoulders. During training, this area can become tight and lead to pain. Tightness in this area can also contribute to pain in the front of the shoulder.

1. To stretch your right arm, reach your right arm across your body keeping it parallel with the floor.
2. Using your left arm, place your left hand on your right elbow.
3. Gently pull your elbow to your chest. You should feel a stretch in the back of your right shoulder.
4. Hold for 30 seconds, then perform on the other side.

Dead Hangs

The final exercise that I encourage people to incorporate after bench pressing is known as a Dead Hang. Like the name suggests, you literally hang from a bar and let gravity do the work. There is a surprising number of benefits to doing the Dead Hang exercise, including:

- Increasing Grip Strength
- Forearm Muscle Growth
- Increasing Shoulder Range of Motion
- Increasing Rotator Cuff Strength
- Spine Decompression

Due to all of these benefits, it is important to incorporate them at the end of your workout.

1. Find a pull up bar and grip it about shoulder width with your palms facing away from your body. Make sure your thumbs are wrapped around the bar.
2. Gripping the bar, slowly allow yourself to hang with your elbows completely straight. Bending your elbows engages muscles and defeats the purpose of the exercise.
3. Make sure your upper body muscles are no longer engaged. Everything should be relaxed.
4. Keep your body in line without swinging and hold for as long as you can.

During this exercise, you want your feet off of the floor so that you are at a full hang. If this is too intense initially, you can do this exercise partially by allowing your feet to touch the floor and unweighting them slightly so that your body is still getting the benefits. I suggest seeing how long you can maintain this position initially and do 3-4 sets of it each time. For example, if you can hold for a maximum of one minute, do sets of 30-40 seconds. After a while you will get stronger and you should re-evaluate yourself to determine if you can hold for longer.

GO BENCH PRESS!

Now that I have gone over a correct warm-up, proper bench press form, and post-lifting injury prevention, you are ready to go bench press. I suggest beginning with just the bar and no additional weight so that you can get every component of the lift down before you start to add weight. When you begin to add weight, make sure it is a weight that you can control and perform pain free. The correct warm-up, technique, and post-exercise injury prevention will not only help you stay pain free, but it will also increase your longevity as a weight lifter.

I hope that you have found this publication beneficial. I wanted to keep it short and sweet to include only the most relevant information for your goals. After you begin to incorporate these strategies into your workout, you should feel comfortable bench pressing while avoiding injury as best as possible. When I began to implement these steps, my bench press felt better and I noticed that I was stronger and more stable when performing the lift. Following these guidelines will put you on a great path to accomplishing your bench press goals. I want to thank you very much for following along and I wish you luck in all of your bench press endeavors!

BONUS CHAPTER:
INCLINE BENCH PRESS

One popular variation of bench pressing – and a personal favorite of mine – is the incline bench press. The incline bench press is beneficial because, when done correctly, it will work and develop more of the upper chest muscles. Compared to the flat bench press, the incline bench press has a similar setup and the following rules still apply:

- Check to see if the bar is even in the rack and not lopsided.
- Generally shoulder width to slightly wider than shoulder width grip.
- Gripping the bar close to the base of your palm with the thumb wrapped around for safety.
- Always make sure your wrists are straight and not bent during all aspects of the lift.
- Keep shoulders back and shoulder blades pinched together for stability.
- Push your chest out for greater chest activation.
- Maintain proper shoulder and shoulder blade position to create the natural arch of the spine. DO NOT OVERARCH.
- Keep feet flat on the floor and shins pointing vertically so that they are perpendicular to the ceiling.

- Make sure that your glutes are engaged and you are driving through the floor but keep your butt on the bench.
- Keep elbows locked straight and begin with the bar over the eyes. Before you descend, have the bar directly over your shoulders.
- Inhale when the bar is descending towards your chest and exhale as the bar moves away from your chest.
- The starting position should be with the bar over your shoulders.
- Maintain a vertical forearm position and prevent the elbows from flaring out during all times. Elbows should be less than 90 degrees away from the side of your body.

Now, you are probably asking about how the bar path should be for incline bench press because I have not included that in the list. This is the main difference between incline and flat bench press and I want to harp on this. Since this exercise focuses more on the upper chest, this is exactly where you want to lower the bar to. To do this safely, you lower the bar from directly over your shoulders to your upper chest. If you want a good mark of where to lower to, aim to touch right below your clavicle, also known as the collar bone. Commonly, you will see people lowering the bar way too low, which puts extreme strain on your shoulders. Remember to make sure that the bar comes down to right below your clavicles and then press it up back to the starting position.

If you maintain a stable shoulder blade position and follow the directions above, you should not have any issue touching the bar to your chest. If you do have difficulty with this, it's okay to not lower it all the way. Like I mentioned before, everyone is different. I know people who prefer not to do this. Play around with the form and find the best fit for you.

REFERENCES

J Fradkin, Andrea & R Zazryn, Tsharni & Smoliga, James. (2009). Effects of Warming-up on Physical Performance: A Systematic Review With Meta-analysis. Journal of strength and conditioning research / National Strength & Conditioning Association. 24. 140-8. 10.1519/JSC.0b013e 3181c643a0.

Kim TW, An DI, Lee HY, Jeong HY, Kim DH, Sung YH. Effects of elastic band exercise on subjects with rounded shoulder posture and forward head posture. *J Phys Ther Sci*. 2016; 28(6): 1733-7.

ABOUT THE AUTHOR

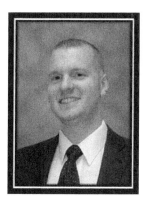

Nicholas Gallo is a board certified Doctor of Physical Therapy. He has helped countless patients in his career and continues to practice Physical Therapy on a full time basis. He is also a cofounder of Physical Therapy 101.

ADDITIONAL RESOURCES

———————

For more information, visit my website at www.physicaltherapy101.net. Here we have resources on various pathologies. This website is continuously updated to provide up to date treatment and is a great resource for practitioners, patients, and prospective Physical Therapists.

Subscribe to my YouTube channel https://www.youtube.com/c/PhysicalTherapy101. Here we produce free treatment videos for patients and healthcare providers. This is also a great visual aid for treatments described above.

I have other publications that you may also find interesting:

Posture Pain: Key Strategies to Stay Pain Free at Your Desk and in Life – I discuss the optimal computer station setup to maintaining ideal posture, exercises to perform to reduce pain, and ways to implement these strategies in other scenarios.

Getting Into Physical Therapy School: 10 Essential Things You Must Do – I systematically outline the process of applying to Physical Therapy School, how to specifically strengthen your application, and beat the competition with key strategies.

P.S. If you have enjoyed this book and found it resourceful, please leave a helpful review on Amazon.

Printed in Great Britain
by Amazon

83020711R00031